Pharmacist Mom

What a Diabetic Needs to Know

Written by: Karen Schindell

Pharmacist

Copyright 2024 by Karen Schindell

Table of Contents

Understanding Diabetes

Introduction

Diabetes is a chronic condition that affects millions of people worldwide, making it crucial to understand its underlying mechanisms, causes, and management strategies. In this chapter, we will delve deeper into the different types of diabetes, explore the role of diet and nutrition in managing blood sugar levels, discuss various monitoring devices and techniques, examine medications commonly prescribed for diabetes management, explore potential complications of the condition, and highlight the importance of emotional well-being in diabetes care. By gaining a comprehensive understanding of diabetes, we can empower ourselves to take control of our health and live fulfilling lives.

Section 1: Types of Diabetes

1.1 Type 1 Diabetes

Type 1 diabetes is an autoimmune disease in which the body's immune system mistakenly attacks and destroys the insulin-producing cells in the pancreas. This results in a significant reduction or complete absence of insulin production, leading to high blood sugar levels. Typically diagnosed during childhood or adolescence, individuals with type 1 diabetes require lifelong insulin therapy. This type of diabetes makes up about 5-10% of diagnosed cases and necessitates careful blood glucose monitoring and insulin administration to maintain stable blood sugar levels.

Recent research has also indicated a potential genetic predisposition for type 1 diabetes, with certain genes increasing the likelihood of developing the condition. However, the exact causes are still not fully understood, and they may involve both genetic and environmental factors. Viral infections, exposure to certain chemicals, and dietary factors have been explored in relation to the development of type 1 diabetes, but further studies are needed to establish definitive links.

1.2 Type 2 Diabetes

The most common form of diabetes is type 2 diabetes, accounting for approximately 90-95% of cases. Unlike type 1 diabetes, type 2 diabetes is often associated with lifestyle factors like obesity and sedentary behavior. In this type, the body either becomes resistant to the effects of insulin, leading to elevated blood glucose levels, or it fails to produce enough insulin to meet the body's needs.

While genetics play a role, factors like excess body weight, poor diet, physical inactivity, and certain ethnic backgrounds significantly contribute to its development.

Emerging evidence suggests that abdominal fat, specifically visceral fat, plays a central role in the development of insulin resistance. This type of fat is metabolically active and releases compounds that impair insulin's actions. Furthermore, chronic inflammation, cellular stress, and dysfunction of specialized cells in adipose tissue, called adipocytes, contribute to the disruption of insulin signaling pathways.

Effective management of type 2 diabetes involves lifestyle modifications, including healthy eating, regular exercise, weight management, and, in some cases, medication or insulin therapy. Losing excess weight, particularly abdominal fat, has been shown to improve insulin sensitivity and glycemic control. Therefore, strategies that focus on promoting weight loss through dietary changes, increasing physical activity, and behavior modifications are vital components of type 2 diabetes management.

1.3 Gestational Diabetes

Gestational diabetes occurs during pregnancy and affects approximately 7% of all pregnancies. It is caused by hormonal changes during pregnancy that impair insulin sensitivity, resulting in elevated blood sugar levels. While it usually resolves after childbirth, women with gestational diabetes have an increased risk of developing type 2 diabetes later in life. It is essential to manage gestational diabetes carefully to prevent complications for both the mother and the baby.

Pregnant women with gestational diabetes need regular monitoring of blood glucose levels and may require dietary modifications, increased physical activity, and/or medication to maintain blood sugar control. A multidisciplinary approach involving obstetricians, endocrinologists, dietitians, and diabetes educators is beneficial to ensure the health and well-being of both mother and baby.

Section 2: Managing Diabetes

2.1 Diet and Nutrition

The role of diet and nutrition in managing diabetes goes beyond simply controlling blood sugar levels. A well-balanced, individualized eating plan can help manage weight, prevent or manage cardiovascular risk factors, maintain optimal blood pressure and cholesterol levels, and improve overall health and well-being.

Consuming a diet rich in whole grains, lean proteins, healthy fats, and a variety of fruits and vegetables is essential for maintaining stable blood sugar levels. Carbohydrates, in particular, have a direct impact on blood sugar levels. Carbohydrate counting, a method of matching insulin doses to the amount of carbohydrates consumed, is an effective way to maintain blood glucose control. Understanding the glycemic index and glycemic load of foods can also assist in determining their impact on blood sugar levels. Additionally, working with a registered dietitian or certified diabetes educator can provide valuable guidance in creating individualized meal plans, taking into account personal preferences, cultural considerations, and overall nutritional needs.

It is important to note that dietary recommendations for diabetes management are not "one size fits all." The nutritional needs and goals may vary depending on the type of diabetes, medication usage, age, sex, activity levels, and overall health status. Regular monitoring of blood sugar levels, along with the guidance of healthcare professionals, enables individuals to make necessary adjustments to their dietary strategies.

2.2 Physical Activity

Regular physical activity is integral to diabetes management, helping improve insulin sensitivity, promote weight loss or maintenance, and enhance overall well-being. Engaging in both aerobic exercises, such as walking, swimming, or cycling, and strength training exercises can have a positive impact on blood sugar control.

Exercise leads to increased glucose uptake by muscles, allowing them to utilize glucose as energy and reduce blood sugar levels. It also enhances insulin sensitivity, allowing the body to use insulin more effectively. Moreover, physical activity helps manage weight, improve cardiovascular health, reduce blood pressure, and lower the risk of developing other chronic conditions associated with diabetes, such as heart disease and stroke.

While physical activity plays a crucial role in diabetes management, it is essential to consider certain factors before starting an exercise regimen. Consulting with healthcare professionals, especially if there are any underlying health concerns, can help determine the most suitable exercise program and precautions to take. Regular monitoring of blood sugar levels, adjusting medications accordingly, and staying hydrated during exercise are important considerations for safe participation. Additionally, individuals with diabetes should be aware of the signs and symptoms of hypoglycemia during and after physical activity, as adjustments in medication or carbohydrate intake may be necessary.

2.3 Monitoring Blood Glucose

Monitoring blood glucose levels is a vital component of diabetes management. By checking blood sugar regularly, individuals can make informed decisions regarding medication dosage, dietary adjustments, and lifestyle modifications. Various monitoring devices, such as glucose meters, continuous glucose monitors (CGMs), and flash glucose monitoring systems, provide accurate and convenient ways to track blood sugar levels.

Glucose meters, commonly used by individuals with diabetes, require a small blood sample obtained through finger pricking. CGMs, on the other hand, provide continuous glucose readings by inserting a small sensor under the skin, eliminating the need for frequent finger pricks. These devices allow for real-time monitoring, detection of trends and patterns, and more comprehensive data for effective diabetes management. Flash glucose monitoring systems provide glucose readings by scanning a sensor worn on the back of the upper arm, providing a snapshot of glucose levels in the interstitial fluid.

Understanding target ranges, interpreting results, and knowing when and how to take corrective action are essential skills for effective self-management. Healthcare professionals play a crucial role in guiding individuals on appropriate monitoring techniques, target levels, and troubleshooting strategies. They can also provide education on how to interpret the results and make informed decisions based on the readings.

Regular monitoring of blood glucose levels allows individuals to identify patterns and trends in their blood sugar levels, helping them make necessary adjustments to their treatment plan. It also enables early detection of high or low blood sugar levels, reducing the risk of complications and allowing for timely intervention.

In addition to monitoring blood glucose levels, individuals with diabetes may need to monitor other parameters, such as blood pressure, cholesterol levels, and kidney function. These additional tests provide valuable information about overall health and help identify potential complications associated with diabetes.

2.4 Medications for Diabetes Management

Medication is an essential tool in managing diabetes, particularly for individuals with type 1 diabetes and some individuals with type 2 diabetes. While lifestyle modifications are the foundation of diabetes management, medications are often necessary to achieve optimal blood sugar control.

For individuals with type 1 diabetes, insulin is the primary medication required. Insulin can be administered through injections or an insulin pump, which delivers insulin continuously throughout the day. The dosage and timing of insulin administration are determined by healthcare professionals based on factors such as blood sugar levels, dietary intake, physical activity, and individual needs.

Type 2 diabetes management may involve various medications, depending on the individual's blood sugar control and overall health. These medications work in different ways to lower blood sugar levels, either by increasing insulin production, improving insulin sensitivity, reducing glucose absorption in the intestine, or slowing down glucose production in the liver. The choice of medication depends on factors such as blood sugar levels, other health conditions, potential side effects, and individual preferences.

In recent years, advancements in diabetes treatment have led to the development of new classes of medications known as incretin-based therapies and sodium-glucose co-transporter 2 (SGLT2) inhibitors. These medications have shown promising results in improving blood sugar control, promoting weight loss, and reducing cardiovascular risk in individuals with type 2 diabetes.

Some more well-known Brand Names of these are: Invovokana®, Farxiga®, and Jardiance®.

But as with any medication, these can have side effects as well. Since one way of working is that they excrete excess sugar via urinating, they tend to cause yeast infections both in women and men.

It's important to note that medication usage may change over time, and adjustments may be needed based on changes in blood sugar levels, overall health status, and response to treatment. Regular communication with healthcare professionals is crucial in determining the most appropriate medication regimen and ensuring optimal diabetes management.

Section 3: Complications of Diabetes

3.1 Acute Complications

Diabetes can give rise to acute complications, which require immediate medical attention. These complications include hypoglycemia (low blood sugar) and hyperglycemia (high blood sugar).

Hypoglycemia occurs when blood sugar levels drop too low. It can be caused by excessive insulin or diabetes medication dosage, delayed or missed meals, increased physical activity, or alcohol consumption without adequate food intake. Symptoms of hypoglycemia include shakiness, dizziness, confusion, irritability, sweating, and in severe cases, seizures or loss of consciousness. Prompt treatment of hypoglycemia typically involves consuming a fast-acting source of glucose, such as fruit juice, glucose tablets, or candy.

Hyperglycemia, on the other hand, occurs when blood sugar levels are elevated. It may be caused by factors such as inadequate insulin dosage, consuming excessive carbohydrates, physical or emotional stress, illness, or medication side effects. Symptoms of hyperglycemia include excessive thirst, frequent urination, fatigue, blurred vision, and slow wound healing. If left untreated, hyperglycemia can lead to diabetic ketoacidosis (DKA) in individuals with type 1 diabetes or hyperosmolar hyperglycemic state (HHS) in individuals with type 2 diabetes. Both DKA and HHS are serious conditions that require immediate medical attention.

3.2 Long-Term Complications

Uncontrolled diabetes can lead to long-term complications that affect various organ systems in the body. These complications develop gradually over time and can significantly impact quality of life and overall health.

Diabetic retinopathy is a condition that affects the blood vessels in the retina, resulting in vision impairment and blindness if left untreated. Regular eye examinations and early detection are essential to manage diabetic retinopathy effectively.

Diabetic neuropathy is nerve damage caused by high blood sugar levels. It commonly affects the feet and legs, causing numbness, tingling, pain, and the loss of sensation. Individuals with diabetes need to pay close attention to foot care, including daily inspections, wearing appropriate footwear, and seeking prompt medical attention for any foot-related issues.

Diabetic nephropathy is kidney damage that occurs due to prolonged exposure to high blood sugar levels. It is a leading cause of end-stage renal disease (ESRD), requiring dialysis or kidney transplantation. Regular monitoring of kidney function through urine testing and blood tests is critical for early detection and appropriate management.

Cardiovascular disease is a major concern for individuals with diabetes, as they have a higher risk of developing heart disease and stroke. Managing blood pressure, cholesterol levels, and maintaining optimal blood sugar control are crucial in reducing the risk of cardiovascular complications.

Other long-term complications associated with diabetes include peripheral arterial disease (reduced blood flow to the limbs), gastroparesis (delayed stomach emptying), erectile dysfunction, and skin conditions. Regular medical check-ups, ongoing monitoring, and maintaining a healthy lifestyle are essential in preventing and managing these complications.

Section 4: Emotional Well-being in Diabetes Care

The emotional well-being of individuals with diabetes is a critical aspect of their overall health. Living with a chronic condition can lead to various emotions, including fear, stress, anxiety, and depression. These emotional challenges can affect diabetes self-management and quality of life.

It is important for individuals with diabetes to have a support system that includes healthcare professionals, friends, family, and diabetes support groups. Support can provide a sense of understanding, encouragement, and guidance. Additionally, seeking professional help from therapists or counselors can help individuals cope with the emotional impact of diabetes and develop adaptive strategies to manage stress.

Self-care practices, such as engaging in enjoyable activities, practicing relaxation techniques, and maintaining a positive mindset, can also contribute to emotional well-being. Regular self-reflection and setting realistic goals can help individuals with diabetes overcome challenges and maintain a sense of control over their condition.

Conclusion

Understanding the different types of diabetes, implementing appropriate lifestyle modifications, regularly monitoring blood sugar levels, utilizing medications effectively, and managing emotional well-being are essential components of diabetes care. With knowledge and proactive self-management, individuals can lead fulfilling lives and effectively navigate the complexities of living with diabetes. It is important to seek support from healthcare professionals, maintain a positive mindset, and stay informed about recent advancements in diabetes management to ensure optimal health and well-being.

Types of Diabetes

Diabetes is a complex and chronic condition that affects millions of people worldwide. While the most common types of diabetes are Type 1 and Type 2, there are also several other types that are less well-known but equally important to understand. This chapter will explore the different types of diabetes and their unique characteristics.

1. Type 1 Diabetes:
Type 1 diabetes, also known as juvenile diabetes or insulin-dependent diabetes, is an autoimmune disease in which the immune system mistakenly attacks and destroys the insulin-producing cells in the pancreas. This results in a complete deficiency of insulin, a hormone necessary for regulating blood sugar levels. Type 1 diabetes is usually diagnosed in childhood or adolescence, but it can occur at any age.

The exact cause of Type 1 diabetes is still unknown, but it is believed to result from a combination of genetic factors and environmental triggers. Some studies suggest that certain viruses, such as enteroviruses, may play a role in triggering the autoimmune response. Type 1 diabetes cannot be prevented, and those affected require daily insulin injections or the use of an insulin pump to manage their blood sugar levels.

Managing Type 1 diabetes requires constant monitoring of blood sugar levels, regular insulin administration, and close attention to diet and physical activity. Technology advancements, such as continuous glucose monitors and insulin pumps, have made it easier for individuals with Type 1 diabetes to manage their condition. However, it is essential to maintain optimal blood sugar control to reduce the risk of long-term complications such as nerve damage, kidney disease, eye problems, and cardiovascular diseases.

   2. Type 2 Diabetes:
Type 2 diabetes is the most common type of diabetes and typically develops in adulthood, although it can also occur in children. It occurs when the body becomes resistant to the effects of insulin or doesn't produce enough insulin to

maintain normal blood sugar levels. Type 2 diabetes is often associated with lifestyle factors such as poor diet, physical inactivity, obesity, and family history.

The development of Type 2 diabetes is influenced by a combination of genetic and lifestyle factors. Individuals with a family history of diabetes, especially in close relatives, have an increased risk of developing the condition. Lifestyle choices, such as sedentary behavior, unhealthy eating habits, and obesity, also contribute to the development of insulin resistance.

Unlike Type 1 diabetes, Type 2 diabetes can often be prevented or delayed through healthy lifestyle changes. These changes include adopting a balanced diet rich in whole grains, fruits, vegetables, lean proteins, and healthy fats; engaging in regular physical activity; maintaining a healthy weight; and avoiding tobacco and excessive alcohol consumption. In some cases, oral medications or insulin injections may be necessary to manage blood sugar levels. Uncontrolled Type 2 diabetes can lead to complications such as heart disease, kidney damage, eye problems, and nerve damage.

3. Gestational Diabetes:

Gestational diabetes is a form of diabetes that develops during pregnancy and usually disappears after delivery. It occurs when the body is unable to produce and utilize enough insulin to meet the demands of pregnancy. Gestational diabetes affects approximately 2-10% of pregnancies worldwide, and the prevalence is increasing due to factors such as obesity and sedentary lifestyles. The hormonal and metabolic changes during pregnancy can contribute to insulin resistance, which leads to increased blood sugar levels. Women who have risk factors such as a family history of diabetes, being overweight or obese, or having previously given birth to a large baby are more likely to develop gestational diabetes.

Managing gestational diabetes is crucial to prevent complications for both the mother and the baby. Regular monitoring of blood sugar levels, following a balanced diet tailored to meet the needs of pregnancy, engaging in regular physical activity, and sometimes using insulin therapy are essential strategies. By effectively managing blood sugar levels, the risk of complications such as preeclampsia, early delivery, and an increased risk of Type 2 diabetes later in life for both the mother and the child can be reduced.

4. LADA (Latent Autoimmune Diabetes in Adults): LADA is a form of diabetes that shares some characteristics of both Type 1 and Type 2 diabetes. It is often misdiagnosed as Type 2 diabetes because it typically affects adults over the age of 30. LADA is an autoimmune condition in which the immune system gradually destroys the insulin-producing cells in the pancreas.

LADA progresses more slowly than Type 1 diabetes, and individuals may not require insulin therapy immediately. However, over time, LADA may progress to a point where insulin treatment becomes necessary. It is important for healthcare providers to differentiate LADA from Type 2 diabetes to provide appropriate treatment options and prevent delays in initiating insulin therapy.

Research suggests that LADA may have a stronger genetic component than Type 2 diabetes, and certain genetic markers have been associated with an increased risk of LADA. Understanding an individual's specific genetic profile is crucial for optimal treatment and management of LADA.

5. MODY (Maturity-Onset Diabetes of the Young): MODY is a rare form of diabetes caused by genetic mutations that affect the beta cells in the pancreas. It usually manifests in early adulthood or adolescence, but it can develop at any age. MODY is characterized by impaired insulin production, and the severity of symptoms can vary based on the specific gene mutation. MODY is often misdiagnosed as Type 1 or Type 2 diabetes, but it requires a different treatment approach. Genetic testing is essential to identify the specific genetic mutation responsible for MODY, as this information can guide treatment decisions and help determine whether oral medications or insulin injections are necessary.

Like other forms of diabetes, managing MODY involves maintaining optimal blood sugar control to prevent short-term symptoms and long-term complications. Lifestyle modifications such as a healthy diet, regular exercise, and maintaining a healthy weight are important factors in managing MODY effectively.

Understanding the different types of diabetes is crucial for effective management and treatment. Each type has its own unique characteristics and may require specific approaches to maintain optimal blood sugar control. Seeking medical guidance and support is essential to ensure an accurate diagnosis and personalized treatment plan. With proper management and a comprehensive approach to care, individuals with diabetes can lead fulfilling lives while reducing the risk of complications associated with the disease.

The Importance of Diet for Diabetics

Maintaining a healthy diet is not only important for overall well-being but is especially crucial for individuals living with diabetes. Diet plays a critical role in the management of diabetes, and often serves as the foundation for treatment. A well-balanced and carefully planned diet can help regulate blood sugar levels, manage body weight, and reduce the risk of complications associated with diabetes.

Diabetes is a complex condition that affects the body's ability to process glucose effectively. When managing diabetes through diet, the primary objective is to maintain stable blood sugar levels. This entails a close monitoring of carbohydrate intake, as carbohydrates have the most significant impact on blood glucose levels. Diabetics must be mindful of the types and amounts of carbohydrates they consume to prevent sharp spikes or drops in blood sugar.

Carbohydrates can be divided into two main categories: simple carbohydrates and complex carbohydrates. Simple carbohydrates, found in refined sugars and processed foods, are quickly digested and absorbed, leading to a rapid increase in blood sugar. Foods such as white bread, sugary snacks, and sweetened beverages fall into this category and should be limited or avoided. On the other hand, complex carbohydrates, found in whole grains, legumes, and vegetables, are digested more slowly, resulting in a gradual rise in blood sugar levels. These foods should be the primary source of carbohydrates for individuals with diabetes.

While carbohydrates require careful consideration, it is also important to focus on consuming adequate amounts of protein and healthy fats. Protein not only helps stabilize blood sugar levels but also promotes satiety and aids in the maintenance of muscle mass. Incorporating lean meats, fish, tofu, and legumes into daily meals can be beneficial. Healthy fats, such as those found in avocados, nuts, seeds, and olive oil, are essential for overall health and can enhance insulin sensitivity. Including these types of fats in moderate amounts can provide long-lasting energy and promote a feeling of fullness.

Portion control is a key aspect of managing diabetes through diet. It is essential to be mindful of the size of each meal and distribute carbohydrate, protein, and fat intake throughout the day. This approach helps prevent blood sugar spikes and promotes better glucose control. Dividing meals into smaller, more frequent portions can also aid in maintaining stable blood sugar levels.

Another important concept in a diabetic diet is the glycemic index (GI), which ranks foods based on how they affect blood sugar levels. Foods with a low GI are digested and absorbed more slowly, resulting in a gradual rise in blood sugar. Examples of low GI foods include whole grains, non-starchy vegetables, and certain fruits. These foods can be incorporated into the diet to maintain consistent blood sugar levels and prevent sudden fluctuations.

Monitoring and understanding the effects of different foods on blood sugar levels is crucial for individuals with diabetes. Regularly testing blood sugar levels after meals and keeping a food diary can help identify patterns and learn how different foods impact glucose levels. By tracking their diet and blood sugar levels, individuals can make adjustments and gain better insight into the foods that work best for their diabetes management.

In addition to managing blood sugar levels, a diabetes-friendly diet can also help address other related health concerns. For instance, individuals with diabetes often experience a higher risk of cardiovascular disease. Incorporating heart-healthy food choices into their diet, such as omega-3 fatty acids from fish and nuts, fiber-rich whole grains, and antioxidant-rich fruits and vegetables, can help improve heart health and reduce the risk of complications.

Furthermore, the diet of individuals with diabetes should also focus on maintaining a healthy weight. Maintaining a healthy weight is beneficial in managing blood sugar levels, improving insulin sensitivity, and reducing the risk of other obesity-related conditions. Alongside a balanced diet, regular physical activity is also crucial for achieving and maintaining a healthy weight. Engaging in regular exercise helps improve insulin sensitivity, promote weight loss, and increase overall cardiovascular fitness.

It is important for individuals with diabetes to work with a healthcare professional or a registered dietitian who specializes in diabetes care to develop a personalized meal plan. A healthcare professional can consider individual needs, preferences, and any other relevant health conditions while creating a comprehensive and effective diet plan.

A healthy diet is not a temporary fix but a lifelong commitment for individuals living with diabetes. With the right approach to diet and the guidance of healthcare professionals, diabetics can successfully manage their condition, improve overall health and well-being, and enjoy a good quality of life.

Choosing the Right Foods for Blood Sugar Control

Instead of solely focusing on the total amount of carbohydrates consumed, it is advisable to opt for complex carbohydrates that are rich in fiber. These complex carbohydrates are digested more slowly, resulting in a gradual release of glucose into the bloodstream and helping to prevent blood sugar spikes.

Whole grains are an excellent source of complex carbohydrates. Unlike refined grains, which have been processed and stripped of their bran and germ, whole grains retain all parts of the grain—endosperm, bran, and germ—providing more fiber, vitamins, minerals, and phytochemicals. Whole wheat bread, brown rice, quinoa, oatmeal, and buckwheat are great examples of whole grains that can be incorporated into a diabetic's diet. Not only do they provide fiber, but they also have a lower glycemic index, meaning they have a less pronounced impact on blood sugar levels compared to their refined counterparts. Choosing whole grains over refined grains is a simple yet powerful step towards better blood sugar control.

Non-starchy vegetables are another important aspect of a diabetic's diet. These vegetables are high in fiber, vitamins, and minerals while being low in carbohydrates and calories. Incorporating a variety of non-starchy vegetables into meals helps maintain a balanced diet while keeping blood sugar levels stable. Dark leafy greens like spinach and kale, cruciferous vegetables such as broccoli and cauliflower, as well as colorful bell peppers and zucchini, are all excellent choices that provide an abundance of nutrients. Including non-starchy vegetables in every meal can enhance satiety, support weight management, and ensure optimal blood sugar control.

Protein plays a critical role in blood sugar regulation as well. Consuming protein-rich foods helps slow down the digestion process, preventing rapid rises in blood sugar levels. Lean meats, such as poultry and fish, are excellent sources of high-quality protein. Fish, especially fatty fish like salmon, trout, and sardines, provide omega-3 fatty acids, which have been shown to reduce inflammation and improve insulin sensitivity. Plant-based proteins like tofu, tempeh, and legumes are also healthy options for diabetics, as they are low in saturated fat and high in fiber. Incorporating protein into meals and snacks can promote satiety, stabilize blood sugar levels, and support overall health.

Healthy fats should also be included in a diabetic's diet. Although fats should be consumed in moderation due to their high caloric density, they can help promote satiety and stabilize blood sugar levels. Opting for heart-healthy fats found in avocados, nuts, seeds, and olive oil can provide essential nutrients and contribute to overall well-being. These monounsaturated and polyunsaturated fats can have positive effects on blood sugar control and reduce the risk of heart disease, a common complication in diabetes. Including a small portion of healthy fats in each meal can add flavor and satisfaction while supporting healthy blood sugar levels.

While it is important to focus on the proper food choices, there are certain foods that diabetics should limit or avoid entirely. Sugary beverages, including soda, fruit juices, and sports drinks, can cause significant blood sugar spikes and should be replaced with water or unsweetened beverages. Processed and refined foods, such as white bread, sugary snacks, and desserts, should also be limited as they are typically high in simple carbohydrates and unhealthy fats. These foods can lead to rapid blood sugar fluctuations and contribute to weight gain, insulin resistance, and various health complications.

It's essential to remember that everyone's dietary needs may vary, and it is recommended to work with a registered dietitian or nutritionist to develop an individualized meal plan. These professionals can provide guidance on portion sizes, carbohydrate counting, and meal timing based on your medication regimen and lifestyle. By collaborating with a healthcare professional, you can create a personalized meal plan that suits your specific needs and goals, ensuring optimal diabetes management and overall well-being.

In conclusion, choosing the right foods for blood sugar control is fundamental for effectively managing diabetes. Prioritizing complex carbohydrates, non-starchy vegetables, lean proteins, and healthy fats while limiting or avoiding sugary beverages and processed foods is key. Incorporating whole grains, non-starchy vegetables, lean meats, plant-based proteins, and heart-healthy fats into your diet can support stable blood sugar levels and provide essential nutrients for overall health. Remember to work with a healthcare professional or nutritionist to tailor a meal plan specifically for you. Empowering yourself with the knowledge and resources to make healthier food choices will enable you to take control of your diabetes and lead a healthier, more balanced life.

Monitoring Blood Glucose Levels

Monitoring blood glucose levels is a crucial aspect of diabetes management. By regularly checking your blood sugar levels, you can understand how well your body is processing glucose and make necessary adjustments to maintain optimal control. This chapter will explore why monitoring blood glucose levels is important and provide insights into the different methods and devices available for monitoring.

To start with, monitoring blood glucose levels provides valuable information about how food, exercise, medication, stress, and other factors affect your blood sugar levels. By tracking your levels before and after meals, you can identify how certain foods impact your blood sugar and make informed choices about meal planning. For example, you may notice that consuming food with high carbohydrate content causes an immediate spike in your blood sugar levels. Over time, this knowledge can guide you in choosing healthier options or adjusting your insulin dosage.

Additionally, monitoring can help you understand the effects of physical activity on your glucose levels, allowing you to adjust your exercise routine accordingly. Regular physical activity is essential for managing diabetes as it helps to lower blood sugar levels and improves insulin sensitivity. By monitoring your blood sugar levels before and after exercise, you can determine if your current activity level is effective or if adjustments need to be made. For example, if your blood sugar levels consistently drop too low during or after exercise, you may need to adjust your insulin dosage or consume a small snack before working out.

Furthermore, monitoring blood glucose levels allows you to identify and manage fluctuations caused by medication. Diabetes medications such as insulin or oral hypoglycemic agents play a crucial role in regulating blood sugar levels. However, individual responses to these medications can vary, and monitoring can help you assess their effectiveness. Regular monitoring can reveal whether a particular medication is adequately controlling your blood sugar levels or if an adjustment is necessary. It is important to work closely with your healthcare provider to ensure that your medication regimen aligns with your blood glucose goals.

Regularly monitoring your blood glucose levels also enables you to detect patterns and trends. By tracking your levels over time, you can identify if your levels are consistently high or low at specific times of the day, making it easier to adjust your medication or meal timings accordingly. For instance, if you consistently experience high blood sugar levels in the morning, you may need to make changes to your medication or revisit your dinner choices. Recognizing these patterns helps you take proactive steps to maintain better control over your blood sugar levels and avoid any potential complications.

This data can also be useful when discussing your diabetes management with your healthcare provider. By sharing your blood glucose monitoring records with your doctor or diabetes educator, they can analyze the trends and provide personalized guidance. They may recommend changes to your medication or insulin regimen, suggest adjustments in your meal plan, or provide strategies to address specific challenges you may be facing. Regular communication and collaboration with your healthcare team are vital in achieving your target blood glucose levels and overall health goals.

There are various methods and devices available for blood glucose monitoring. The traditional method involves using a lancing device to obtain a small drop of blood from your fingertip and applying it to a test strip inserted into a blood glucose meter. The meter then measures your blood sugar level and displays it on the screen. This method provides accurate results and is widely used. However, it requires regular finger pricks, which some people find uncomfortable or inconvenient.

Another option for monitoring involves continuous glucose monitoring (CGM) systems. These systems consist of a tiny sensor inserted under the skin that measures glucose levels in the fluid between the cells. The sensor transmits real-time glucose readings to a receiver or a smartphone app, allowing you to monitor your levels without frequent finger pricks. CGM systems provide continuous data and can help you visualize glucose patterns throughout the day. This technology has proven to be advantageous in identifying trends, providing alerts for high or low blood sugar levels, and aiding in adjusting insulin dosages.

Some blood glucose meters also offer features like insulin dose calculators, memory storage, and connectivity to mobile apps, making it easier to track and analyze your data. These additional features can be helpful for individuals who prefer a more comprehensive monitoring experience or those who are keen on incorporating technology into their diabetes management routine.

It is essential to follow proper technique and guidelines when monitoring blood glucose levels. Ensure that you wash your hands thoroughly before testing to avoid contaminants that may affect the accuracy of the readings.

Follow the instructions provided with your device or consult your healthcare provider for guidance on how often to monitor your blood sugar levels and when to take action based on the results. Remember, accuracy and consistency are critical to making informed decisions about your diabetes management.

Monitoring your blood glucose levels is not just about numbers; it is about understanding your body and making informed decisions. By regularly tracking and analyzing your levels, you can strive for better control and reduce the risks associated with diabetes. Remember to work closely with your healthcare team to interpret your results and make necessary adjustments to your diabetes management plan.

In the next chapter, we will explore the different types of blood glucose monitors available in the market and their features to help you choose the one that suits your needs best. We will delve into the considerations for selecting a blood glucose monitor, such as accuracy, cost, ease of use, and compatibility with your lifestyle. Additionally, we will discuss advances in technology and the future of blood glucose monitoring, offering insights into potential developments that may further enhance diabetes management for individuals worldwide.

Different Types of Blood Glucose Monitors

Different Types of Blood Glucose Monitors

In today's age of technological advancements, there are multiple types of blood glucose monitors available for individuals with diabetes to choose from. These monitors play a vital role in helping individuals manage their blood sugar levels effectively and make informed decisions about their diabetes care. To better understand the diverse options available, let's delve into the different types of blood glucose monitors in greater detail:

1. Fingerstick Glucose Meters: Fingerstick glucose meters are the most commonly used and widely accessible type of blood glucose monitors. These portable devices have been a staple in diabetes management for many years. They work by obtaining a small blood sample, typically from the fingertip, which is then placed onto a test strip inserted into the meter. The meter analyzes the sample and provides a digital reading of the current blood glucose level. Modern fingerstick glucose meters have evolved to include several convenient features, including memory storage to track

past readings, data transfer capabilities for sharing information with healthcare professionals, and advanced data analysis to identify trends and patterns in glucose levels.

Advances in fingerstick glucose meters have also focused on improving accuracy and ease of use. Many new models require smaller blood samples, reducing discomfort for individuals with sensitive fingertips. Some devices also feature alternate site testing options, allowing blood samples to be taken from the forearm or palm instead of the fingertip. This provides flexibility for individuals who prefer to avoid fingerstick testing or require alternative testing sites due to conditions such as peripheral neuropathy.

2. Continuous Glucose Monitoring (CGM) Systems: CGM systems have revolutionized the way individuals with diabetes monitor their blood glucose levels. These advanced devices provide real-time glucose monitoring throughout the day and night, offering a comprehensive view of glucose fluctuations. A small sensor, usually inserted under the skin on the abdomen or arm, measures glucose levels in the interstitial fluid. The readings are then wirelessly transmitted to a receiver or a smartphone app. One example of a CGM is the Dexcom G6®. Keep in mind that blood glucose monitors are constantly being upgraded and the current model may change.

CGM systems offer a multitude of benefits beyond just glucose monitoring. They provide valuable insights into glucose trends and patterns, allowing individuals to understand how their blood sugar levels change in response to various factors like meals, exercise, and stress. This data empowers individuals to make proactive adjustments to their diabetes management plan, optimizing their blood sugar control. CGM systems also offer customizable alerts for low and high blood sugar levels, helping individuals avoid severe hypoglycemic or hyperglycemic events.

3. Flash Glucose Monitoring (FGM) Systems: FGM systems, also known as "glucose sensing technology," provide individuals with an alternative and convenient way to monitor their blood glucose levels. These systems share similarities with CGMs but offer distinct features. Like CGMs, FGM systems consist of a small sensor attached to the skin, which measures glucose levels in the interstitial fluid. However, unlike CGMs, FGM systems do not require frequent calibration or the use of a separate receiver.

FGM systems are known for their simplicity and ease of use. Instead of continuous glucose readings, individuals using FGM systems can conveniently scan the sensor with a compatible reader or smartphone app to obtain instant glucose readings. This non-invasive method of glucose monitoring eliminates the need for routine fingerstick testing, making FGM systems a convenient option for individuals who dislike or find fingerstick tests challenging. FGM systems also provide insights into glucose trends and patterns, allowing individuals to monitor their blood sugar levels without interruption while still obtaining valuable information to inform their diabetes management. An example of a machine with this technology at the time of the writing of this is the FreeStyle Libre 2®.

4. Insulin Pump Integrated Systems: Insulin pump integrated systems combine the functionalities of an insulin pump and a continuous glucose monitor. These systems allow individuals with diabetes to manage both their insulin delivery and their glucose monitoring from a single device. The insulin pump integrates with a subcutaneous glucose sensor, which provides continuous glucose readings. By continuously monitoring glucose levels, the pump can automatically adjust insulin delivery based on the individual's needs.

Insulin pump integrated systems offer greater convenience and precision in diabetes management. The continuous monitoring provided by the glucose sensor enables the pump to make real-time adjustments to insulin delivery, reducing the risk of hypoglycemia or hyperglycemia. Some systems even have advanced algorithms that can predict impending high or low blood sugar levels and adjust insulin delivery preemptively. By closely intertwining insulin delivery and glucose monitoring, pump integrated systems offer individuals with diabetes a more streamlined and synchronized approach to their diabetes care.

When considering which blood glucose monitor to choose, it's essential for individuals with diabetes to consult with healthcare professionals. Factors such as personal preferences, lifestyle, budget, and the level of glucose monitoring required should be taken into account to determine the most suitable monitor for each individual's specific needs.

Remember, consistent and accurate blood glucose monitoring is crucial for effective diabetes management. The different types of blood glucose monitors available today offer a wide range of features that can assist individuals in gaining better control over their blood sugar levels and ultimately improving their overall quality of life.

Medications for Diabetes Management

Managing diabetes involves a multi-faceted approach that includes lifestyle changes, diet modifications, and, in many cases, the use of medications. Medications for diabetes management aim to control blood sugar levels, improve insulin sensitivity, and prevent complications associated with the disease. In this chapter, we will explore the different types of medications commonly used in the treatment of diabetes.

1. Oral Medications:

a) Metformin:
Metformin is considered the first-line choice for treating type 2 diabetes due to its effectiveness and safety profile. It helps lower blood glucose levels primarily by reducing glucose production in the liver and increasing insulin sensitivity in the body's tissues. Metformin does not stimulate insulin release from the pancreas. It is typically well-tolerated and has a low risk of hypoglycemia. However, some individuals may experience gastrointestinal

side effects such as stomach upset, diarrhea, and nausea. It is important to take metformin with meals to minimize these side effects.

b) Sulfonylureas:

This class of drugs stimulates the pancreas to release more insulin, helping to lower blood sugar levels. Sulfonylureas have been widely used for many years and are available in different forms, including glipizide, glyburide, and glimepiride. They can effectively control blood sugar levels, but they do pose a risk of hypoglycemia, particularly in older adults and those with impaired kidney function. Sulfonylureas may also lead to weight gain and should be used cautiously in individuals with a history of sulfa allergies.

c) Dipeptidyl peptidase-4 (DPP-4) inhibitors:

DPP-4 inhibitors work by increasing insulin release and decreasing the hormone glucagon, which typically raises blood sugar levels. Examples of DPP-4 inhibitors include sitagliptin (Januvia®) , saxagliptin (Onglyza®), and linagliptin (Tradjenta®). These medications are generally well-tolerated and have a low risk of hypoglycemia. However, they may cause side effects such as upper respiratory tract infections and joint pain. DPP-4 inhibitors are a suitable choice for individuals who require better blood sugar control without weight gain or the risk of hypoglycemia.

d) Thiazolidinediones (TZDs):

TZDs, such as pioglitazone (Actose®) and rosiglitazone (Avandia®), improve insulin sensitivity in target tissues, allowing the body to use insulin more effectively. They may also reduce glucose production in the liver. TZDs can be particularly useful in individuals with insulin resistance and those with a high risk of cardiovascular disease. However, TZDs have been associated with an increased risk of heart failure and may cause weight gain, fluid retention, and bone fractures. Regular monitoring of liver enzymes and heart function is necessary for individuals taking TZDs.

2. Injectable Medications:

a) Insulin:

Insulin is a crucial hormone that helps regulate blood sugar levels. For individuals with type 1 diabetes or advanced type 2 diabetes, insulin is essential. It can be delivered through injections or insulin pumps. Various types of insulin are available, classified based on their onset, peak, and duration of action. Insulin therapy aims to mimic the body's natural insulin production and is tailored to individual needs. The dosage of insulin might fluctuate throughout the day based on factors such as meals, physical activity, and stress levels. Side effects of insulin can include hypoglycemia and weight gain. Proper injection technique and regular monitoring of blood sugar levels are vital for optimal insulin therapy.

b) Glucagon-like peptide-1 (GLP-1) receptor agonists:
GLP-1 receptor agonists are injectable medications that mimic the action of naturally occurring GLP-1 hormones. They stimulate insulin release, inhibit glucagon secretion, slow down digestion, and promote a feeling of fullness. Examples of GLP-1 receptor agonists include exenatide (Byetta®, Bydureon®), liraglutide (Victoza®, Saxenda®) and dulaglutide (Trulicity®). These medications are typically used in individuals with type 2 diabetes who have difficulty managing their blood sugar levels with oral medications alone. GLP-1 receptor agonists have shown cardiovascular benefits and can lead to weight loss. However, they may cause side effects such as nausea, vomiting, and an increased risk of pancreatitis.

3. Combination Medications:

Some medications combine two or more classes to provide a synergistic effect in controlling blood sugar. For instance, metformin may be combined with a sulfonylurea or a DPP-4 inhibitor to enhance its effects. Combination medications offer convenience by reducing the number of pills and potential side effects associated with multiple medications. Certain combination medications also provide extended-release formulations, allowing for once-daily dosing. It is essential to work with a healthcare professional to determine the most appropriate combination therapy based on individual needs and medication tolerability.

It is important to note that diabetes management is not solely reliant on medications. Lifestyle modifications such as adopting a healthy diet, engaging in regular physical activity, and managing stress are integral parts of an effective treatment plan. Medications should be seen as tools to aid in blood sugar control while addressing the underlying causes of diabetes. Always follow your healthcare provider's instructions regarding medication usage, dosage, and potential side effects. Regular monitoring of blood sugar levels is also critical to ensure the effectiveness of medication and make any necessary adjustments to the treatment plan.

Remember: Combining medication management with a comprehensive approach that addresses all aspects of diabetes will yield the best results and help individuals lead fuller, healthier lives. Consult with your healthcare team to develop an individualized treatment plan that suits your needs and goals.

Following Your Doctor's Prescription

Following Your Doctor's Prescription: Taking Charge of Your Diabetes Management

Managing diabetes requires a collaborative effort between the patient and the healthcare provider. Your doctor plays a crucial role in helping you understand and control your diabetes. This chapter will guide you on how to effectively follow your doctor's prescription and recommendations while empowering you to take charge of your diabetes management.

Building a Trustworthy Partnership

Establishing a relationship of trust with your doctor is of utmost importance. Your doctor should be someone who listens to your concerns, answers your questions, and supports you throughout your diabetes journey. Open and honest communication is vital for effective diabetes management. If you feel hesitant or uncomfortable with your doctor, consider seeking a second opinion or finding a healthcare provider who better suits your needs.

Understanding Your Medications

When your doctor prescribes medication, it is essential to fully comprehend the purpose, dosage, and timing. Different medications have various effects on blood sugar levels, and following the instructions precisely can significantly impact your diabetes control. Take the time to ask your doctor about any potential interactions with other medications or supplements you are taking. Educate yourself about the medications prescribed to you so you can be proactive in managing possible side effects and preventing dangerous interactions.

For some people with diabetes, insulin may be necessary to maintain optimal blood sugar control. Insulin can be prescribed in various forms, such as rapid-acting, short-acting, intermediate-acting, and long-acting. Your doctor will determine the appropriate type(s) of insulin for your specific needs and help you understand how and when to administer them. It is crucial to learn the correct injection technique and storage requirements for insulin to ensure its effectiveness.

Other non-insulin medications, such as oral antidiabetic drugs, may also be prescribed. These medications work in different ways to help regulate blood sugar levels, either by stimulating insulin production, improving insulin sensitivity, or reducing glucose production in the liver.

Understanding how these medications work and adhering to your prescribed regimen will optimize their benefits.

Developing Healthy Lifestyle Habits

While medications play a crucial role in diabetes management, they are not the sole solution. Your doctor will likely also recommend lifestyle modifications to help you better control your diabetes. The two most important aspects are diet and exercise.

Your doctor may refer you to a registered dietitian who specializes in diabetes care. They will work with you to design a personalized meal plan that considers your food preferences, calorie requirements, and blood sugar management goals. Adopting a well-balanced diet with appropriate portion sizes can help regulate your blood sugar levels, promote weight management, and minimize the risk of complications.

In addition to meal planning, monitoring your carbohydrate intake is a key aspect of diabetes management. Carbohydrates affect blood sugar levels more significantly than other macronutrients, so understanding how different foods impact your glucose levels is essential. Your doctor or dietitian can teach you how to read food labels, estimate carbohydrate content, and create a meal plan that maintains stable blood sugar levels throughout the day.

Physical activity is equally important in diabetes management. Regular exercise improves insulin sensitivity, helps control weight, and boosts overall well-being. Consult with your doctor before starting any exercise regimen to ensure it aligns with your specific health needs. They can provide guidelines tailored to your abilities and any complications you may have. Aim for a mix of aerobic exercises (such as brisk walking, swimming, or cycling) and strength training activities to reap the maximum benefits.

Sticking to Your Medication Routine

Creating a consistent routine for taking your medications is vital for adequate blood sugar control. Set reminders on your phone, use pill organizers, or associate medication intake with specific daily activities to establish a habit. Consistency will reduce the likelihood of missed doses or accidentally taking double doses. If you encounter any challenges in following your medication routine or experience side effects, promptly consult your doctor. They can guide you on how to best manage these issues and may consider adjusting your medication if necessary.

Regular Check-ups for Optimal Care

Regular visits to your doctor are essential to monitor your progress and adjust treatment plans as needed. Maintaining a schedule of check-ups ensures that your diabetes management remains effective and that any changes in your health are promptly addressed. During these appointments, your doctor will review your blood sugar control, assess the impact of medications and lifestyle changes, and order relevant laboratory tests. Prepare for these visits by keeping track of your blood sugar levels, any symptoms or difficulties you encounter, and questions you may have. Sharing this information with your doctor allows for a more comprehensive understanding of your diabetes management, leading to more effective treatment decisions.

Empowering Yourself through Education

While your doctor serves as a valuable source of information, it is essential to become proactive in your diabetes management. Educate yourself about diabetes, its complications, and the latest advancements in treatment. Understanding the science behind diabetes and its impact on your body can help you make informed decisions regarding your lifestyle, medication, and overall well-being.

Attend diabetes education programs or support groups to connect with others in similar situations. Learning from their experiences and sharing your own challenges can provide valuable insights and emotional support. These programs often cover topics such as blood sugar monitoring, healthy eating habits, physical activity, and medication management. Take advantage of online resources, books, and reputable websites to deepen your understanding. However, always be cautious of unreliable sources and consult with your healthcare team if you have any doubts or questions.

Your active involvement and commitment to your health are crucial for successful diabetes management. Equip yourself with knowledge, stay informed about emerging research, and consistently strive to improve your lifestyle habits. Collaborate with your healthcare team, involve your loved ones in your diabetes management, and reach out for support when needed.

Remember, by following your doctor's prescription, attending regular check-ups, and actively participating in your own care, you are taking charge of your diabetes management. Empowered with knowledge and supported by your healthcare team, you can lead a fulfilling and healthy life despite your diabetes diagnosis.

Recognizing and Managing Low Blood Glucose

Low blood glucose, also known as hypoglycemia, can occur in individuals with diabetes when their blood sugar levels drop below normal. It is important to recognize and manage low blood glucose promptly to prevent complications and ensure overall well-being. In this chapter, we will discuss the signs and symptoms of low blood glucose and provide strategies for managing this condition effectively.

Signs and Symptoms of Low Blood Glucose:

1. Sweating: Excessive sweating, particularly clammy skin, is a common symptom of low blood glucose. When blood sugar levels are low, your body might respond by releasing stress hormones, causing increased sweating. This can be a helpful signal to recognize when your blood sugar is dropping. If you suddenly find yourself sweating for no apparent reason, it could be a sign that your blood sugar level is too low.

2. Shakiness and Weakness: Feeling shaky or weak, as if your muscles are trembling or lacking strength, can be an indication of low blood glucose. This symptom occurs when your brain is not receiving enough glucose, its main energy source. It may be accompanied by an overall sense of fatigue and difficulty concentrating. Some individuals also experience a feeling of internal trembling, which can be distressing. Recognizing these signs can prompt you to take action and treat your low blood glucose promptly.

3. Hunger: Sudden intense hunger, even shortly after eating, can be an indicator of low blood glucose. When blood sugar levels drop, your body sends signals to your brain, triggering hunger hormones. You may experience strong cravings or a feeling of emptiness in your stomach. This type of hunger is different from normal hunger and is often accompanied by other low blood glucose symptoms. If you find yourself feeling ravenously hungry even after a meal, it might be a sign that your blood sugar levels are low.

4. Dizziness and Lightheadedness: Feeling dizzy or lightheaded is another common symptom of low blood glucose. The brain relies on a steady supply of glucose for proper functioning. When blood sugar levels drop, the brain experiences a temporary lack of fuel, leading to these unsettling sensations. You may feel unsteady on your feet or have difficulty maintaining your balance. Hallmark signs of dizziness or lightheadedness can serve as a cue to check your blood sugar levels.

5. Irritability and Mood Changes: Low blood glucose can affect your mood and mental state. Studies have shown that even mild hypoglycemia can lead to irritability, mood swings, and cognitive impairment. This happens because glucose is essential for optimal brain function, and when levels drop, it can impact your overall mood, making you easily agitated, irritable, or anxious. Additionally, confusion and difficulty concentrating can also arise due to insufficient glucose reaching the brain. Recognizing these emotional and cognitive changes can help you better manage your low blood glucose.

Managing Low Blood Glucose:

1. Immediate Treatment: It is crucial to act promptly when experiencing symptoms of low blood glucose. Consume a fast-acting carbohydrate source, such as glucose tablets, fruit juice, or regular soda, to raise your blood sugar levels quickly. It is important to monitor your blood sugar closely after treatment to ensure it returns to a safe range. Remember to follow up with a snack or meal that contains a combination of carbohydrates and protein to help stabilize your blood glucose levels. Delaying or ignoring the treatment of low blood glucose can lead to a further drop in blood sugars and more severe symptoms.

2. Regular Blood Sugar Monitoring: Monitoring your blood glucose levels regularly is an essential part of managing low blood glucose episodes. By regularly checking your levels, especially before and after meals, physical activity, and at bedtime, you can identify patterns and take proactive measures to prevent future episodes. Your healthcare provider might recommend a specific frequency of testing based on your individual needs. It is also essential to keep a record of your readings to share with your healthcare team during check-ups. This information can guide adjustments in your diabetes management plan, insulin dosage, or medications.

3. Adjust Medication or Insulin Dosage: If you are consistently experiencing low blood glucose, consult your healthcare provider. They may need to adjust your medication or insulin dosage to better manage your blood sugar levels. Changes in medication or insulin routines should always be done under professional guidance to avoid any unwanted risks. Your healthcare team will take into account factors such as your type of diabetes, overall health, physical activity, and diet before making any adjustments.

4. Snacking: Eating regular, well-balanced meals and snacks throughout the day can help prevent low blood glucose. Ensure that your meals and snacks contain a combination of carbohydrates, protein, and healthy fats to provide sustained energy and prevent sudden drops in blood sugar. Carbohydrates are the main nutrient that affects blood

sugar levels; however, pairing them with protein or fat can help slow down the absorption of glucose, providing a more stable and prolonged source of fuel. Consider working with a registered dietitian or diabetes educator to develop a personalized meal plan that meets your specific needs.

5. Communicate with Others: It is crucial to inform your family, friends, and colleagues about your condition and educate them on how to recognize and respond to low blood glucose episodes. Provide them with information on the signs and symptoms of low blood glucose and what actions to take if you require assistance. This can provide a safety net of support and assistance when needed. Additionally, wearing a medical ID bracelet or necklace that identifies you as having diabetes can be valuable in case of an emergency.

6. Exercise Precautions: Regular physical activity is an essential component of diabetes management; however, it can also increase the risk of low blood glucose if not properly managed. It is important to monitor your blood glucose levels before, during, and after exercise. If your blood sugar levels are lower than desired, it may be necessary to have a snack or adjust your carbohydrate intake before exercising. Keep sources of fast-acting carbohydrates readily available during physical activity to treat any potential low blood glucose episodes.

Recognizing and managing low blood glucose requires constant vigilance and proactive measures. By staying aware of your body's signals, regularly monitoring your blood glucose, and following your healthcare provider's recommendations, you can successfully navigate and manage low blood glucose episodes. Remember, maintaining a healthy lifestyle, managing stress levels, and adhering to your diabetes management plan are also essential in minimizing the occurrence of low blood glucose.

Recognizing and Managing High Blood Glucose

High blood glucose, also known as hyperglycemia, is a common problem among individuals with diabetes. It occurs when there is an excessive amount of glucose in the bloodstream and can lead to various complications if not properly managed. This chapter will delve into the symptoms, causes, and strategies for recognizing and effectively managing high blood glucose levels.

Recognizing the Symptoms of High Blood Glucose:

1. Increased thirst: When blood glucose levels are high, the body tries to eliminate the excess glucose through increased urine production. This leads to dehydration and subsequently increased thirst. It is important to stay hydrated by drinking adequate amounts of water throughout the day.

2. Frequent urination: Excess glucose in the bloodstream causes the kidneys to work harder to filter and remove it, resulting in increased urine production. This can lead to more frequent trips to the bathroom, especially during the

night. If you notice a significant increase in urination frequency, it is essential to consult your healthcare provider.

3. Fatigue and weakness: High blood glucose levels can hinder the body's ability to effectively use glucose for energy. Without sufficient energy, a person may experience general fatigue and weakness, hindering their daily activities. Feeling consistently exhausted despite adequate rest could be a sign of high blood glucose levels.

4. Blurred vision: Elevated blood glucose can cause fluid to be pulled from the lenses of the eyes, affecting their ability to focus properly. This can result in blurred vision and difficulty seeing clearly. If you experience sudden changes in your vision, it is crucial to consult with your healthcare provider.

5. Increased hunger: Despite having high blood glucose levels, the body's cells may not be receiving sufficient glucose for energy. This can trigger an increase in hunger levels, making individuals feel the need to eat more frequently. It is important to make wise dietary choices during these episodes and prioritize nutrient-dense foods to help manage hunger cravings effectively.

Causes of High Blood Glucose:

1. Insufficient insulin: In individuals with type 1 diabetes, high blood glucose is usually caused by a lack of insulin production. Insulin is necessary to transport glucose from the bloodstream into the cells for energy. In type 2 diabetes, it can occur due to insulin resistance, where the body's cells become less responsive to insulin, or insufficient insulin production. Insulin therapy or other glucose-lowering medications are often prescribed to counteract this issue.

2. Inadequate medication or insulin dosage: Failing to take prescribed medications or using an incorrect dosage can result in high blood glucose levels. It is crucial to adhere to the medication regimen prescribed by your healthcare provider to help control blood glucose levels effectively. Regular communication with your healthcare team will ensure that your medications are appropriately adjusted when needed.

3. Poor dietary choices: Consumption of high-carbohydrate or sugary foods can cause blood glucose levels to spike. These foods are rapidly broken down into glucose, leading to a surge in blood sugar levels. It is important to make informed dietary choices and strive for a well-balanced meal plan that includes whole grains, lean proteins, healthy fats, and ample fruits and vegetables. Portion control and carbohydrate counting can also help regulate blood glucose levels.

4. Lack of physical activity: Regular exercise plays a vital role in blood glucose management. It helps lower blood glucose levels by increasing insulin sensitivity, enabling the body's cells to effectively use glucose for energy. A sedentary lifestyle can contribute to high blood glucose levels, so it is important to incorporate physical activity into your daily routine. Consult with your healthcare provider before starting any exercise regimen to ensure it is safe and suitable for your specific needs.

Managing High Blood Glucose:

1. Monitor blood glucose levels: Regularly checking blood glucose levels, as prescribed by your healthcare provider, helps identify high values promptly. This allows for timely intervention and adjustments to your management plan as needed. Self-monitoring of blood glucose using a glucometer or continuous glucose monitoring systems can provide valuable insights for managing blood glucose levels effectively.

2. Take prescribed medications: It is crucial to take medications or administer insulin as prescribed by your healthcare provider to help control blood glucose levels. These medications work in various ways, such as increasing insulin production, facilitating glucose utilization, or reducing glucose production in the liver. Following the prescribed medication regimen is important as it aids in maintaining stable blood glucose levels.

3. Modify your diet: Consulting a registered dietitian who specializes in diabetes care can help develop a customized meal plan that balances carbohydrate intake and promotes blood glucose control. They will guide you in portion control, limiting sugary foods, and including more whole grains, lean proteins, healthy fats, and vegetables. It is crucial to spread carbohydrate intake evenly throughout the day and pay attention to the glycemic index of foods consumed, as it can impact blood glucose levels differently.

4. Engage in physical activity: Regular exercise helps lower blood glucose levels by increasing insulin sensitivity and improving glucose uptake by the muscles. Aim for at least 150 minutes of moderate-intensity aerobic activity per week, such as brisk walking, cycling, or swimming, along with strength training exercises at least two days a week. However, it is essential to consult with your healthcare provider before starting any exercise regimen to ensure it is safe and suitable for your specific needs.

5. Stay hydrated: Drinking plenty of water helps prevent dehydration caused by increased urination associated with high blood glucose levels. Aim to consume at least eight glasses (64 ounces) of water per day, and adjust this amount based on factors such as climate, exercise, and

individual needs. Avoid sugary drinks and alcohol, as they can further elevate blood glucose levels.

6. Follow your healthcare provider's advice: Regularly visiting your healthcare provider and following their recommendations for blood glucose monitoring, medication adjustments, and lifestyle changes is essential in managing high blood glucose levels effectively. They will provide guidance on setting target blood glucose ranges and help you understand the appropriate steps to take when your blood glucose levels are not within the desired range.

It is important to remember that everyone's response to high blood glucose levels may vary. Additionally, additional factors like stress, illness, and medication changes can influence blood glucose levels. It is crucial to work closely with your healthcare provider to develop an individualized plan for managing and preventing high blood glucose episodes. With proper education, proactive management, and a team approach, individuals with diabetes can successfully maintain stable blood glucose levels and reduce the risk of complications.

Potential Complications of Diabetes

Living with diabetes involves careful management and ongoing monitoring to keep blood sugar levels in check. While proper management can significantly reduce complications, it is important to be aware of the potential complications that can arise if diabetes is not properly controlled. This chapter will explore some of the most common complications associated with diabetes and provide in-depth information on their prevention and management.

1. Cardiovascular Complications:
Diabetes increases the risk of developing cardiovascular diseases such as heart attacks, strokes, and peripheral artery disease. High blood sugar levels can damage blood vessels, leading to the formation of plaque, which can cause blood clots or narrowed arteries. This process is known as atherosclerosis and can occur in any blood vessel, including those supplying the heart, brain, or limbs.

To prevent cardiovascular complications, it is crucial to maintain optimal blood sugar, blood pressure, and cholesterol levels. This can be achieved through lifestyle changes such as following a healthy diet, regular exercise, smoking cessation, and, if necessary, medications as prescribed by your doctor. A diet rich in fruits, vegetables, whole grains, lean proteins, and healthy fats can help lower cholesterol levels and reduce the risk of plaque formation. Moderate-intensity aerobic exercises like walking, swimming, or cycling for at least 150 minutes per week, along with strength training exercises, can improve cardiovascular health. Regular check-ups and screenings for cardiovascular risk factors, such as EKGs, stress tests, and lipid profiles, are also essential.

2. Diabetic Retinopathy:

Diabetic retinopathy is a complication that affects the eyes. It occurs when high blood sugar levels damage the blood vessels in the retina, leading to vision problems and even blindness if left untreated. Retinopathy can progress through different stages, starting with mild non-proliferative retinopathy to more severe proliferative retinopathy.

To prevent or manage diabetic retinopathy, regular eye exams, at least once a year, are crucial. Early detection allows for timely interventions, such as laser treatment or injections, to prevent vision loss. Maintaining stable blood sugar levels is vitally important, as it has been shown to slow down the progression of retinopathy. Blood pressure control and avoiding smoking are also essential in protecting against diabetic retinopathy. Effective blood pressure control, with a target of less than 130/80 mmHg, can help minimize the damage to retinal blood vessels. Additionally, managing other risk factors such as high cholesterol and kidney disease is important.

3. Diabetic Neuropathy:

Diabetic neuropathy is a condition that affects the nerves and can lead to numbness, tingling, pain, or weakness in the hands and feet. It can also affect various organs, causing digestive issues, urinary problems, and sexual dysfunction. Diabetic neuropathy is primarily caused by high blood sugar levels, but other factors such as inflammation, genetics, and lifestyle choices can contribute to its development and progression.

To prevent or manage diabetic neuropathy, it is crucial to maintain stable blood sugar levels through proper diabetes management. Targeting an HbA1c level of less than 7% is recommended by the American Diabetes Association as it has shown to reduce nerve damage. Regular check-ups with a healthcare professional are important for early detection and prompt management of symptoms. Medications such as anticonvulsants, antidepressants, and pain relievers may be prescribed to help alleviate discomfort and prevent further nerve damage. Good foot care is essential as diabetic neuropathy increases the risk of foot infections and ulcers, which can lead to amputations if not properly managed.

4. Kidney Disease (Diabetic Nephropathy):
Diabetic nephropathy is a potentially serious complication that affects the kidneys. High blood sugar levels can damage the blood vessels in the kidneys, leading to impaired kidney function and even kidney failure. Other factors such as high blood pressure and family history can further increase the risk of developing diabetic nephropathy.

To prevent or slow down the progression of kidney disease, it is vital to regularly monitor kidney function through urine tests and blood tests. Annual measurement of urinary albumin-to-creatinine ratio (UACR) helps detect early changes in kidney function. Blood pressure control is crucial, as high blood pressure can further damage the kidneys. Medications such as ACE inhibitors or ARBs may be prescribed to help protect kidney function. It is also important to adopt a healthy lifestyle, including a balanced diet with limited sodium intake and regular physical activity. Limiting dietary protein to 0.8g/kg/day, if necessary, may be advised to reduce the workload on the kidneys.

5. Increased Risk of Infections:

Diabetes weakens the immune system, making individuals more susceptible to infections. Skin infections, urinary tract infections, and respiratory infections can occur more frequently and be more severe in individuals with diabetes. High blood sugar levels create an environment in which bacteria and fungi can thrive, leading to increased susceptibility to infections.

To prevent infections, individuals with diabetes should maintain good hygiene practices, including frequent handwashing. Proper management of blood sugar levels is crucial, as it helps strengthen the immune system. Consistently achieving target blood sugar levels lowers the risk of infections. Regular vaccinations, such as the flu vaccine and pneumonia vaccine, are also recommended to reduce the risk of infections. It is important to promptly treat any infections that arise with appropriate medications, as untreated infections can lead to serious complications.

6. Foot Complications:

Diabetes can cause nerve damage and poor blood flow to the feet, making them more prone to infections, ulcers, and even amputations. Peripheral neuropathy, a type of nerve damage common in diabetes, can cause numbness or loss of sensation, making it difficult to detect injuries or infections.

Reduced blood flow further impairs wound healing and increases the risk of infections.

To prevent foot complications, individuals with diabetes should check their feet daily for any signs of injury, infections, or abnormalities. It is important to wash the feet daily with lukewarm water and mild soap, making sure to dry them thoroughly, especially between the toes. Applying moisturizer to prevent dry skin is recommended, but it should not be applied between the toes. Wearing properly fitted shoes and socks can help prevent foot injuries. Regular visits to a podiatrist are recommended for proper foot maintenance and early detection of any problems. It is also crucial to maintain stable blood sugar levels, as high blood sugar can exacerbate nerve damage and impair circulation. Blood pressure control, smoking cessation, and regular exercise can further reduce the risk of foot complications.

In conclusion, awareness of potential complications is essential for individuals living with diabetes. By implementing proper diabetes management strategies, including regular check-ups, blood sugar control, a healthy lifestyle, and adherence to medical advice, it is possible to prevent or minimize the impact of these complications. Remember, early detection and intervention can

significantly improve outcomes and enhance the overall quality of life for people with diabetes.

Living a Healthy Life with Diabetes

Living a Healthy Life with Diabetes

Living with diabetes can be challenging, but with the right knowledge, strategies, and support, it is possible to lead a healthy and fulfilling life. This chapter will delve deeper into various aspects of living with diabetes, providing valuable information to help individuals manage their condition effectively and maintain optimal health.

1. Healthy Eating: A crucial aspect of managing diabetes is adopting a healthy and balanced diet. This involves understanding the impact of different food groups on blood sugar levels and making informed choices. While carbohydrates are the main factor affecting blood sugar, it's important to consider the quality and quantity of carbohydrates consumed. High-fiber carbohydrates, such as whole grains, legumes, and vegetables, digest more slowly and have a lower impact on blood sugar levels. Counting carbohydrates and portion control are useful strategies for managing blood sugar. It's also important to consider the glycemic index (GI) of foods, as foods with a

higher GI can cause a quicker rise in blood sugar levels. However, it's essential not to solely focus on carbohydrates, but also include lean proteins, heart-healthy fats, and a variety of fruits and vegetables to ensure a well-rounded, nutrient-rich diet.

2. Regular Exercise: Physical activity is not only beneficial for overall health but also plays a pivotal role in diabetes management. Engaging in regular exercise helps improve insulin sensitivity, lowers blood sugar levels, aids in weight management, and reduces the risk of cardiovascular complications. In addition to aerobic exercises like walking, jogging, or cycling, it's beneficial to incorporate strength training exercises that target major muscle groups twice a week. Strength training helps increase lean muscle mass, which can improve insulin response and overall metabolic health. Flexibility exercises, such as yoga or stretching, promote joint mobility and relaxation. It's important to find activities that are enjoyable and sustainable, as adherence to exercise routines is key for long-term success.

3. Blood Sugar Monitoring: Regularly monitoring blood sugar levels is essential for managing diabetes effectively. This involves using a blood glucose monitor to check blood sugar at various times throughout the day. In addition to pre-meal and post-meal blood sugar checks, individuals may benefit from occasional monitoring at other times, such as before and after exercise, during illness, or in response to

specific symptoms. Continuous glucose monitoring (CGM) systems are also available for more comprehensive and real-time monitoring. By diligently tracking blood sugar levels, individuals can identify patterns and make necessary adjustments to their diet, exercise, and medication regimen. It's important to develop a personalized monitoring routine in consultation with healthcare professionals.

4. Medication Management: For some individuals with diabetes, medication may be necessary to manage blood sugar levels effectively. It's crucial to work closely with healthcare professionals to understand the various types of diabetes medications available and their respective benefits and potential side effects. Common medications include metformin, sulfonylureas, DPP-4 inhibitors, GLP-1 receptor agonists, SGLT-2 inhibitors, and insulin. Each medication has unique mechanisms of action and may be prescribed based on an individual's specific needs and health profile. It's important to take medications as prescribed, follow recommended dosages, and be aware of any necessary precautions or interactions with other medications. Frequent communication with healthcare professionals helps ensure medication regimens are optimized for individual needs.

5. Emotional Well-being: Living with diabetes can sometimes bring about emotional challenges such as stress, anxiety,

and depression. It's essential to recognize and address these emotions to maintain overall well-being. Engaging in stress management techniques such as deep breathing exercises, mindfulness meditation, or practicing relaxation techniques can help regulate stress levels. Seeking support from loved ones, joining support groups, or working with a mental health professional can also play a significant role in managing emotional well-being. Developing positive coping strategies, setting realistic goals, and celebrating personal achievements are powerful tools in coping with the emotional aspects of living with diabetes.

6. Diabetes Care Team: Building a strong multidisciplinary diabetes care team is vital for comprehensive diabetes management. This team typically includes healthcare professionals such as primary care physicians, endocrinologists, dietitians, diabetes educators, and pharmacists. Collaborating with this team ensures that individuals receive the necessary guidance and support to manage diabetes effectively. Regular check-ups and consultations that include comprehensive assessments of blood sugar control, medication adjustments, and overall health monitoring help track progress and address any concerns or challenges that may arise. Education and self-advocacy also play crucial roles in maximizing the benefits of a diabetes care team.

7. Preventing Complications: Managing diabetes well can significantly reduce the risk of developing complications. Regular check-ups, routine screenings, and maintaining a healthy lifestyle are key in preventing complications such as heart disease, kidney disease, nerve damage, and vision problems. Regular eye exams, including comprehensive dilated eye exams, can detect early signs of diabetic retinopathy. Annual or more frequent check-ups with healthcare professionals can help monitor kidney function through urine and blood tests. Managing blood pressure and cholesterol levels, as well as avoiding tobacco use, are important in minimizing the risk of cardiovascular complications. Regular dental check-ups are also important, as diabetes increases the risk of gum disease. It's vital to collaborate with healthcare professionals to establish a comprehensive preventive care plan tailored to individual needs.

8. Adjusting to Diabetes: Coming to terms with a diabetes diagnosis can be challenging emotionally and mentally. However, with time and support, it is possible to adjust to this new reality. Educating oneself about diabetes and staying up-to-date with latest research and treatment options is empowering. It's important to understand the impact of different lifestyle choices, such as diet, exercise, stress management, and medication adherence, on overall health and diabetes management. Engaging in meaningful activities, pursuing hobbies, or joining support groups for individuals with diabetes can provide a sense of community and support. Setting achievable goals and celebrating personal achievements are powerful tools in building resilience and maintaining a positive outlook.

By adopting a healthy lifestyle, regularly monitoring blood sugar levels, effectively managing medications, addressing emotional well-being, collaborating with a diabetes care team, and focusing on preventive care, individuals with diabetes can lead vibrant and fulfilling lives. Diabetes does not define a person but rather presents an opportunity to make positive choices for long-term health and overall well-being. Through self-care, education, and support, individuals can navigate their diabetes journey with confidence and embrace every aspect of life with vitality.

About The Author

Karen Schindell

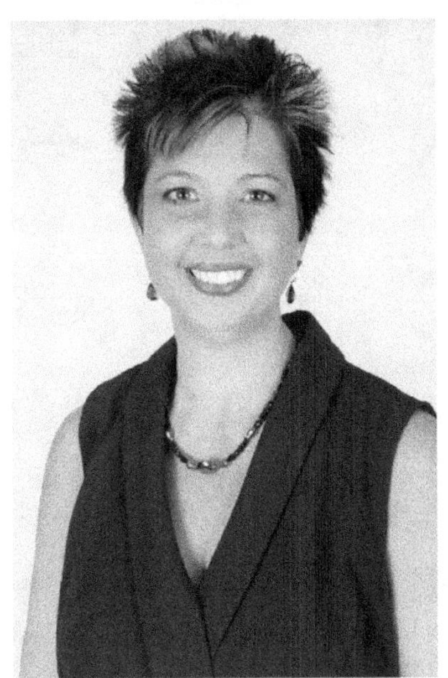

Karen has previously written two children's books under her previous married name (Karen Toliver). *Timmy and Tammy The Sea Turtles Adventures* and *Timmy and Tammy The Sea Turtles Tarpon Springs Adventures.* These books are fun and educational.

Karen is a pharmacist of over 30 years and has a passion of educating. After Educating patients for so long, she has decided to venture out and put that education in writing to try to make it easier for people to understand medication in general.

Being a Florida native, Karen has more recently moved to Kentucky to be near her children and grandbabies to enjoy her family and the beauty of another state has to offer. I hope you enjoy what life has to offer!

Karen